The Ultimate No-Weight Workout

Finally, A Solution For A Great Workout Without The Weights

Lee L. Boyce

The Ultimate No-Weight Workout: Finally, A Solution For A Great Workout Without The Weights

This book was self-published with the amazing help of <u>Self-Publishing Made Easy Now!</u> [1] . You can grab a free copy of the checklist that started my journey here: <u>FREE Self-Publishing Checklist</u> [2] .

[1] https://selfpublishingmadeeasynow.com/xpjv
[2] https://selfpublishingmadeeasynow.com/free_checklist

Table of Contents

1 - Introduction

No weights? No problem.

One of the most common alibis for people who miss working out is that they don't have time to hit the gym or they don't want to spend money on exercise equipment and free weights. Although exercise aids can enhance the experience, they're really not that necessary for someone to have a good full body workout at home or any place desired.

This ebook will show you how you can get that full body strength training without the use of specialized exercise equipment, specifically free weights. You'll be working the upper body muscles which include the chest, back, shoulders, and arms and also the lower body like your thighs, buttocks, and calves. And all of these without using free weights.

Whether your goal is to build a bit of muscle, lose those extra pounds or just simply tone up, these exercises will help you reach your goal.

2 - The Chest

The bench press is still the best exercise in building chest muscles. But using this routine, you'll be toning up those pectorals all in the comfort of your own home. The best workout for your chest, without using weights, is the good old pushup. You might say it's not challenging but you'll change your mind after going through these exercises.

Standard pushup

Begin by lying face down on the floor and your hands directly under the shoulders. Keep your back straight so that the shoulders and the feet form a rigid, straight line.

Pushing with your arms, slowly and steadily lift the torso while keeping the back and legs straight and rigid. Keep doing this until the arms are straight, then slowly lower down the body by bending your arms until they form a 90-degree angle. That would be one repetition.

For beginners, you may start by putting your knees on the floor while doing the standard pushup. This reduces the body weight that you should lift up.

The standard pushup works out the whole chest and should

be the first pushup routine you should be familiar with before moving on to more advanced variations.

Incline pushup

This is similar to the standard pushup, but you need to elevate the upper body using a chair, desk, or bench. Make sure that the furniture doesn't move to avoid injuries.

Lying face down with the hands on the chair and positioned a little wider than shoulder-width. Your feet should also be a hip-width apart and your toes on the floor.

Do the same motion as the standard pushup but when going down, your chest should be just a few inches from the chair. The incline pushup works out your lower and side chest muscles. This is also an easier variation of the pushup because when you are inclined, you use less body weight for resistance.

Elevated pushup

Use the same chair or bench you used in the inclined pushup. Get on the floor using the standard pushup position but this time, place your feet on the chair instead of the ground. You should use a sturdy chair that can support your weight. For added stability, place the chair against the wall.

Do the same motion as you would with the standard pushup. You'll find this a bit more challenging because you'll be pushing more body weight than compared to doing the standard or the inclined pushup.

The elevated pushup works out your upper chest muscles and shoulders.

Advanced pushup variations

The gorilla pushup – Do a basic pushup but do it rapidly so you launch your upper body off the ground, and then clap or slap your chest before returning the hands to the starting position.

Wide pushup – You can widen the position of your hands when doing a standard pushup. This will engage more of the side chest muscles.

Narrow pushup – Position your hands nearer together while doing the pushup motion. This exercise engages more of the inner chest muscles.

3 - The Back

This is the biggest muscle group in your body and having strong back muscles can make a lot of physical work easier. They're also great to have when you need to wear that tank top or that muscle shirt on the beach. Again, if you want really huge back muscles, you should consider using free weights. But if your goal is just to tone up your core back muscles, these exercises are all you need.

Hip Hinge

The hip hinge is the most basic exercise you can do to tone up your back muscles. You simply crease at your hips and flex your torso forward then go back to straight, standing position. But even a simple exercise like the hip hinge can be ruined by poor execution.

You should check for alignment before you begin the exercise. This is best done with a mirror. The ankles, hips, shoulders, and ears should be vertically aligned. This would be the starting position.

Place the hands on the hips. Bend forward by creasing in the hips and maintaining a straight back and until the torso comes parallel to the ground. Slowly straighten up until you're back to the starting position.

The hip hinge is all about alignment and control. Don't rush your movements.

Reverse Snow Angels

Instead of lying flat on your back like you did as you make those snow angels during winter, you'll lie face down and flat on your belly. Do this on the carpet or use a mat for added comfort.

With the palm of your hands facing the ground, place the arms at the side of your torso while keeping the weight in the legs and hips evenly distributed.

Do not let your palms touch the ground. Slowly move the arms in an arching motion until your hands touch, keeping the arms straight the whole time. Yes, like making a snow angel. Slowly go back to the starting position, again without letting your arms touch the floor.

Locust

This is a more advanced weight-less back exercise, but this will activate all the muscles on your back. It was derived from a yoga position and will also work your legs and arms.

Start by lying down on your belly with the arms at the side and the legs straight. Rest your forehead on the floor and keep the palms up.

Slowly lift your head, chest, arms, and the legs and look at the ceiling. Balance on your abdominal area while raising the legs as high as you can.

Slowly go back to the starting position.

4 - The Biceps

The upper arm consists of the biceps and the triceps. Triceps are also worked when doing pushing exercises like pushups and dips. Developing or strengthening the bicep muscles without weights can be difficult but it can surely be done.

Let's look first at the anatomy of a bicep exercise. Basically, in order to develop your bicep muscles, you need to do a curling motion wherein you raise your lower arm towards your shoulders. This engages the bicep muscles but to keep it challenged, you need to incorporate some resistance.

Towel Curls

For this exercise, you'll need a bath towel. Roll it up lengthwise so it forms a thick rope then fold it in half. Sit on a chair then place a leg in the middle of the folded tower. Hold each end of the towel by gripping tightly with each hand.

Now slowly pull the ends of the towel up towards your shoulders without using your leg muscles. The weight of your leg then becomes the resistance for this exercise. The weight of the leg alone can prove to be a challenge for beginners and to add even more resistance, push away using your leg as you pull up the towel.

This exercise imitates doing barbell curls and is great for developing your biceps.

Arm Resistance Curls

So, you can't find a towel to do your bicep exercises? No problem. You can imitate a bicep concentration curl on one arm using the other arm as resistance. This routine is usually done by bodybuilders either as a contest pose or as a warm-up before they go on stage.

You can start by either sitting down on a chair or standing up. The arm being exercised should have its palm up and is placed at the side. Using the other arm, clasp your hands and slowly lift the arm on the side towards the shoulder. As you do this, push with the other arm to provide some resistance. The difficulty of this exercise can be varied by how much resistance you provide with the other arm.

Chin Up

OK. You might say I might be cheating because I'll be recommending an equipment for this exercise since it requires a pull-up bar. Well, you will still be using your body weight for this exercise. Also, you can buy a pull-up bar and put it on a door. It shouldn't cost you that much. This equipment is also versatile since you can do other exercises with it that can strengthen your back and abdominals.

Chin ups incorporate the curling motion as you pull yourself up and try to touch the bar with your chin. Start by gripping the bar firmly with your palms facing your body. The grip should also be shoulder width. Keeping your body straight, slowly pull your body up using your biceps and back muscles until your chin touches the bar. Slowly go back to the starting position.

This exercise is considered an advanced routine because you'll be lifting up your whole-body weight. You can begin with a bit of cheating by stepping on a chair and helping the pull-up motion by pushing down with your feet. Do this until you are able to do a chin up without the chair.

5 - The Triceps

Triceps actually compose a bigger part of your upper arms than biceps do. As the name implies, it's composed of three muscles and is generally used for pushing motion. You use the triceps when you do pushups, which also develop your chest muscles.

There are quite a number of triceps exercises you can do without using free weights but some of them will require equipment. These are routines you can do at home.

Narrow Pushup

Remember the narrow pushup in a previous chapter? That same exercise is actually also great for developing your triceps. Using a narrow grip when doing a pushup incorporates less of the chest muscles and more of the triceps muscles. This is a more difficult variation of the pushup since you'll be relying more on your triceps to push your body off the floor and triceps are generally weaker than chest muscles because they are smaller.

You can do some variations on the narrow pushup routing like putting one of the arms a bit farther away from the inner chests. This is great for challenging an arm or blasting through plateaus. You can also place a couple of thick books under one hand while doing the narrow grip pushup.

You can also do a diamond pushup. This is more difficult than a regular narrow pushup because the positioning of the hands will target your triceps muscles even more. With your index fingers and thumbs, you form a diamond and place it under your chest as you lie face down on the floor. Do the normal pushup motion. You'll feel more burn on your triceps using this variation. Remember to keep your back straight throughout the exercise.

The pushup is a versatile exercise since it can engage more than one muscle group. Variation and volume is the key.

6 - Legs

The muscles on your thighs form the biggest muscle group in your body. These muscles keep you upright when you are standing up and also helps move you around. Evolution did this, so you can walk, run, and jump.

Because a lot of movements are dependent on the legs, they are the easiest to challenge even without using free weights. Again, using free weights can help build bigger leg muscles but you don't need them if all you want is a great and challenging leg workout. Working the legs also engage the other muscles like the buttocks, the hamstrings, and the calves. It is important to wear knee sleeves that can provide the best support and compression.

These exercises will give you the best overall leg workout without the use of free weights.

Squats

The squat is the most common exercise for the legs. It's too common that most people tend to do it improperly. Some people even skip the squat since they say they do it almost every day when sitting down and standing up. But the foundation of all those lower-body workouts is the humble squat. Doing the squat routine can determine how you run, walk, lunge, or jump.

Start by standing with your feet shoulder width apart or wider. Lift your arms up to your front and hold them straight with your palms facing down. Some people would prefer crossing their arms over their shoulders. Holding your arms on the front helps you keep your balance while you do the squat.

Bend your legs on the knees slowly while keeping your back straight and looking straight in front of you. The feet should also lay flat on the floor throughout the exercise. Keep bending your legs until the thighs are parallel to the ground. Slowly stand up keeping the back straight until you're back to the starting position. That would be one repetition.

You might think it's too easy, but when you focus on doing squats for much more than ten repetitions, you'll find the real meaning of a leg day. The squat also works out your lower back, your buttocks, your hamstrings, and your calves.

For variety, you can widen your stance even more. By doing this, you'll engage a lot more of your inner leg muscles. Don't forget to keep your back straight and the width of your stance should be no more than what you are comfortable with or you'll risk injury.

Lunge

Lunges are the next best exercise for your legs, and again, they can effectively be done without using free weights. A lunge is actually a squat, but instead of using both legs, you'll only be using one while the other one stabilizes your pose.

Begin by standing with your legs a shoulder-width apart. Your arms should point down and at your sides. Using one leg, step back then both of your knees to form a 90-degree angle. Pause at this position so you can check if you have the proper form. The shin on the front leg should be vertical and the knee should not pass the toe. Be mindful of your posture by making sure that the torso is vertical and tall. Most people have a tendency to lean forward while doing the lunge. This will put extra strain on your back.

Using a slow, controlled motion, push with the leg on your front by driving your heel to the floor. Go back to the starting position and do the same motions with the other leg.

Glute Bridge

You've seen this move in countless exercise videos and although this exercise also effectively works out your buttocks, it also engages your upper leg muscles. The glute bridge is also recommended for those who cannot do a proper squat or lunge due to physical restraints.

Begin by lying down with your back flat on the floor. With your feet, a shoulder-width apart, bend your knees until they form a 90-degree angle. This will be your starting position.

Slowly push your heels down into the floor while raising your hips up. Do this until your torso is parallel to your thighs then squeeze your glutes and keep your abdomen tight to prevent arching. The shins should also be vertical. Slowly lower your back and go back to the starting position.

For variety, you can use a chair or a Swiss exercise ball to place your feet on. This will engage the thigh muscles and the glutes more.

Step Up

The step up is a very effective yet very low-risk exercise that you can do for your legs or the lower body in general. You can also incorporate this into your routine if you feel that one of your legs is weaker than the other.

You'll be needing a chair or a bench for this exercise. Start by placing a foot on the elevated platform and push down as you stand up straight. Make sure you are not hinging at your hips or leaning forward. Keep your body straight and vertical throughout the motion.

Single Leg Calf Raise

Your calves stabilize your legs as you walk, run, or simply stand up. It's one of the more worked out muscles in your body so growing or developing it can be challenging since it's used to daily torture. You can incorporate more resistance without using free weights by using only one leg.

Stand up straight and lift one of your legs up by bending on the knees. If you can't do this without wobbling, hold on to a chair or a door. Remember to use the least assistance as possible in maintaining your balance. Your goal is to challenge that calf.

Lift yourself up by pushing down with the ball of your foot until you can feel your calf tightening up. Go back to starting position. The idea here is to do the exercise until failure before you switch to the other foot.

7 - Conclusion

Having no free weights or specialized equipment should not be an excuse for not having a full body workout. You don't even have to go to the gym, spend money on gym memberships, or buy your own equipment. You can use your own body weight as resistance to tone or build muscles.

The idea here is variation and volume. You should vary your exercise routines to avoid plateaus. And since you'll be using your body weight for resistance, you should aim for volume. Most of the exercises here should be done until failure. That means until you can't do another repetition anymore. You can then take a minute or two of rest then begin again.

Happy exercising!

Thank You

As we reach the end of this book, I want to say thanks for reading this book.

I want to get this information out to as many people as possible. If you found this book helpful, I would greatly appreciate you leaving me a review. This helps others find the book as well.

This book was self-published with the amazing help of <u>Self-Publishing Made Easy Now!</u> [3] . You can grab a free copy of the checklist that started my journey here: <u>FREE Self-Publishing Checklist</u> [4] .

[3] https://selfpublishingmadeeasynow.com/xpjv
[4] https://selfpublishingmadeeasynow.com/free_checklist

Disclaimer

will any legal responsibility or blame be held against the publisher for any reparation, damages, or monetary loss due to the information herein, either directly or indirectly.